The Vibrant Keto Vegetarian Diet Cooking Book

Don't Miss Amazingly Delicious Smoothies Recipes to Enjoy Every Moment of Your Day

Skye Webb

Table of contents

Chocolate Bread Pudding

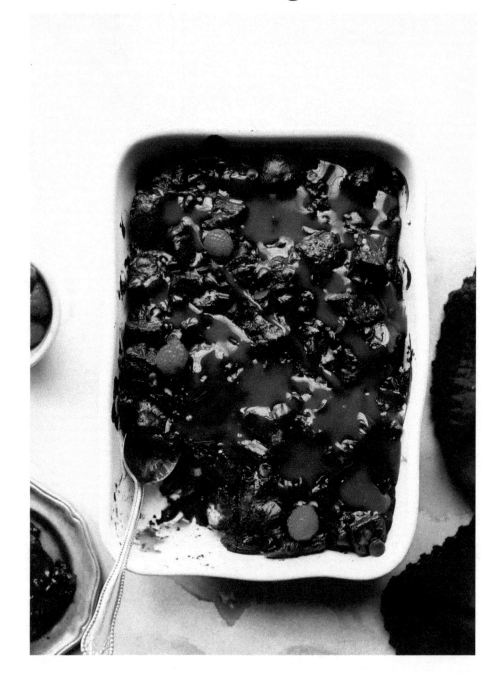

Preparation Time: 40 Minutes Servings: 6

Ingredients:

4 cups white bread cubes

2 cups unsweetened almond milk

2 cups vegan semisweet chocolate chips

½ cup chopped pecans or walnuts

¾ cup granulated natural sugar

¼ cup unsweetened cocoa powder

1 tablespoon vegan butter

1   teaspoon pure vanilla extract

½ teaspoon salt

Directions:

1.   Oil a baking tray that will fit in your Instant Pot.

2.   Melt 1 and 2/3 of the chocolate chips with 1.5 cups of the almond milk.

3.   Spread the bread cubes in your Instant Pot, sprinkle with nuts, and the remaining chocolate chips.

4.   Warm the remaining almond milk in another saucepan with the sugar, cocoa, vanilla, and salt.

5.   Combine the cocoa mix with the chocolate chip mix and pour it over the bread.

6.   Seal your Instant Pot and cook on Beans for 30 minutes.

7.   Depressurize naturally.

Mango Rice Pudding.

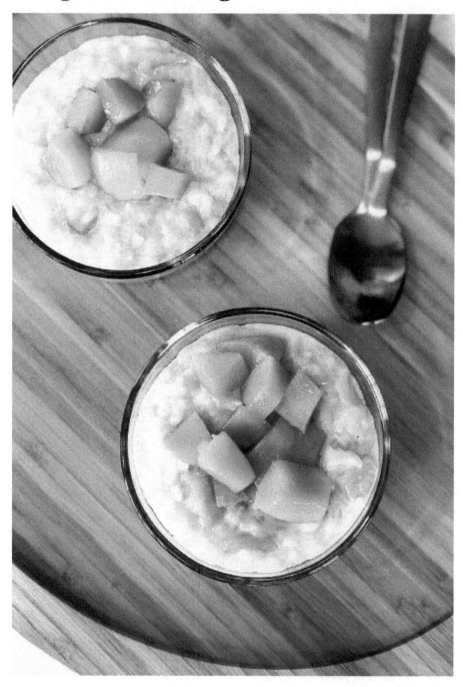

Preparation Time: 35 Minutes Servings: 6

Ingredients:

2   (14-ouncecans unsweetened coconut milk

2 cups unsweetened almond milk, plus more if needed

1 cup uncooked jasmine rice

½ cup granulated natural sugar, or more to taste

1 large ripe mango, peeled, pitted, and chopped

1 teaspoon coconut extract

1 teaspoon pure vanilla extract

¼ teaspoon salt

Directions:

1.   Spray the Instant Pot insert with cooking spray.

2.   Add the milks and bring to a boil.

3.   Add the rice, sugar, and salt, seal, and cook on Rice.

4.   Depressurize quickly and stir in the extracts and mango.

5.   The pudding will thicken as it cools.

Tapioca With Apricots.

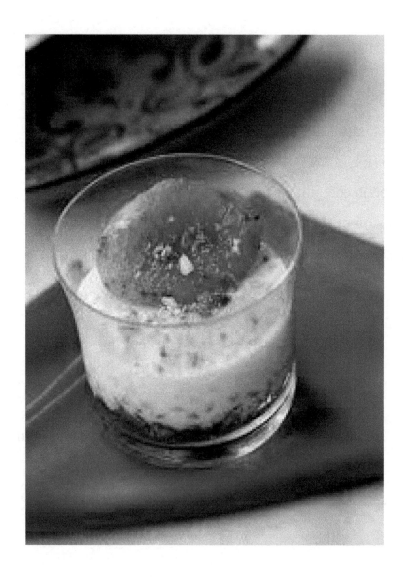

Preparation Time: 25 Minutes Servings: 4

Ingredients:

2½ cups unsweetened almond milk

½ cup chopped dried apricots

⅓ cup small pearl tapioca

⅓ cup granulated natural sugar

¼ cup apricot preserves

1 teaspoon pure vanilla extract

Directions:

1.   Spray the inside of your Instant Pot with cooking spray.

2.   Put in the tapioca, sugar, almond milk, and apricots.

3.   Seal and cook on Stew for 12 minutes.

4.   Release the pressure fast.

5.   In a bowl combine the preserve and vanilla.

6.   Add the mixture to your tapioca and reseal your Instant Pot.

7.   Leave to finish in its own heat.

8.   Serve hot or cold.

Poached Pears In Ginger Sauce.

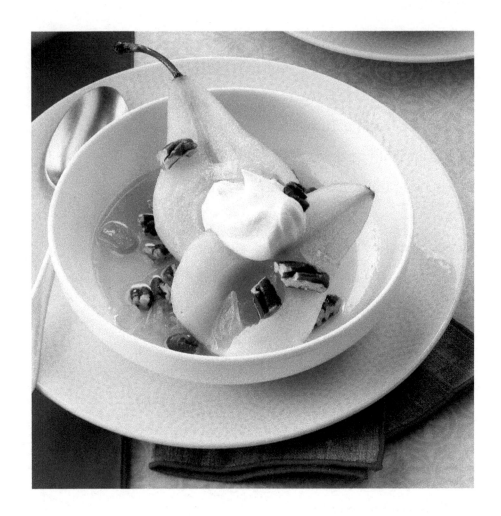

Preparation Time: 25 Minutes Servings: 6

Ingredients:

2½ cups white grape juice

6 firm ripe cooking pears, peeled, halved, and cored

¼ cup natural sugar, plus more if needed

6 strips lemon zest

½ cinnamon stick

2 teaspoons grated fresh ginger

Juice of 1 lemon

Pinch of salt

Directions:

1.   Warm the grape juice, ginger, lemon zest, salt, and sugar until blended.

2.   Add the cinnamon stick and the pears.

3.   Seal and cook on Stew for 12 minutes.

4.   Take the pears out.

5.   Add lemon juice and more sugar to the liquid.

6.   Cook with the lid off a few minutes to thicken.

7.   Serve.

Baked Apples.

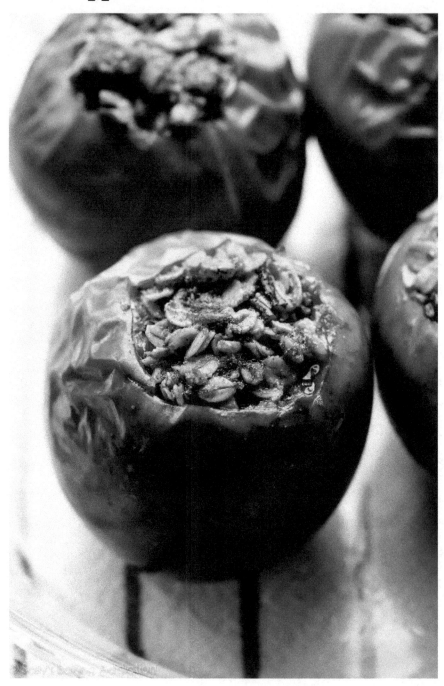

Preparation Time: 35 Minutes Servings: 6

Ingredients:

6 large firm Granny Smith apples, washed

½ cup naturally sweetened cranberry juice

⅓ cup sweetened dried cranberries

⅓ cup packed light brown sugar or granulated natural sugar

¼ cup crushed, chopped, or coarsely ground almonds, walnuts, or pecans

Juice of 1 lemon

½ teaspoon ground cinnamon

Directions:

1.   Core the apples most of the way down, leaving a little base so the stuffing stays put.

2.   Stand your apples upright in your Instant Pot. Do not pile them on top of each other! You may need to do two batches.

3.   In a bowl combine the sugar, nuts, cranberries, and cinnamon.

4.   Stuff each apple with the mix.

5.   Pour the cranberry juice around the apples.

6.   Seal and cook on Stew for 20 minutes.

7.   Depressurize naturally.

Maple & Rum Apples.

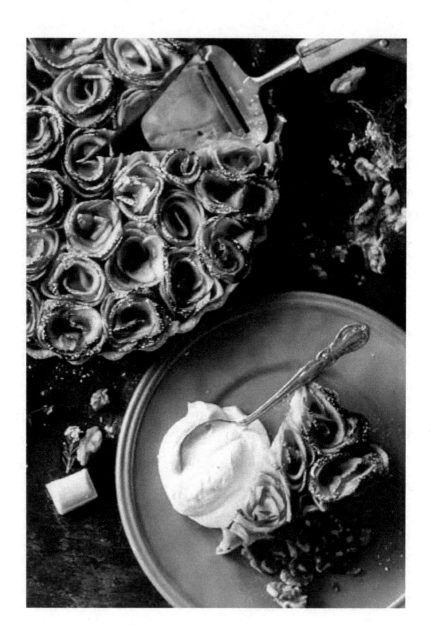

Preparation Time: 25 Minutes Servings: 6

Ingredients:

6 Granny Smith apples, washed

½ cup pure maple syrup

½ cup apple juice

⅓ cup packed light brown sugar

¼ cup golden raisins

¼ cup dark rum or spiced rum

¼ cup old-fashioned rolled oats

¼ cup macadamia nut pieces

1 teaspoon ground cinnamon

½ teaspoon ground nutmeg

Juice of 1 lemon

Directions:

1.   Core the apples most of the way down, leaving a little base so the stuffing stays put.

2.   Stand your apples upright in your Instant Pot. Do not pile them on top of each other! You may need to do two batches.

3.   In a bowl combine the oats, sugar, raisins, nuts, and half the nutmeg, half the cinnamon.

4.   Stuff each apple with the mix.

5.   In another bowl combine the remaining nutmeg and cinnamon, the maple syrup, and the rum.

6.   Pour the glaze over the apples.

7.   Seal and cook on Stew for 20 minutes.

8.   Depressurize naturally.

Pumpkin & Chocolate Loaf.

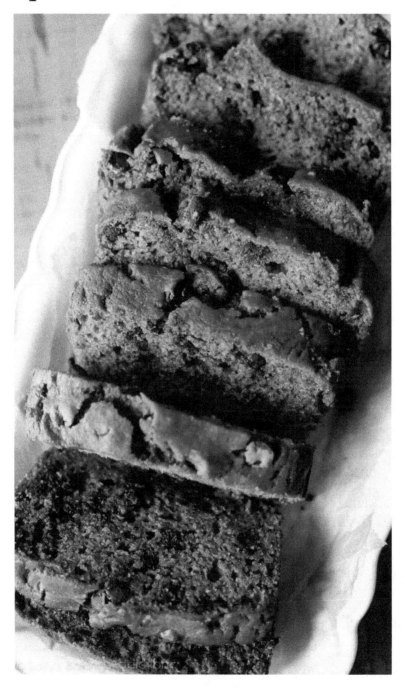

Preparation Time: 15 Minutes Servings: 8

Ingredients:

1¾ cups unbleached all-purpose flour

1 cup canned solid-pack pumpkin

½ cup packed light brown sugar or granulated natural sugar

½ cup semisweet vegan chocolate chips

¼ cup pure maple syrup

2 tablespoons vegetable oil

2 teaspoons baking powder

1 teaspoon pure vanilla extract

½ teaspoon salt

½ teaspoon ground cinnamon

¼ teaspoon ground allspice

¼ teaspoon ground nutmeg

Directions:

1.   Lightly oil a baking tray that will fit in the steamer basket of your Instant Pot.

2.   In a bowl, combine the flour, baking powder, baking soda, salt and spices.

3.   In another bowl combine the pumpkin, maple syrup, sugar, vanilla, and oil.

4.   Stir the wet mixture into the dry mixture slowly until they form a smooth mix.

5.   Fold in the chocolate chips.

6.   Pour the batter into your baking tray and put the tray in your steamer basket.

7.   Pour the minimum amount of water into the base of your Instant Pot and lower the steamer basket.

8.   Seal and cook on Steam for 10 minutes.

9.   Release the pressure quickly and set to one side to cool a little.

Cheesecake

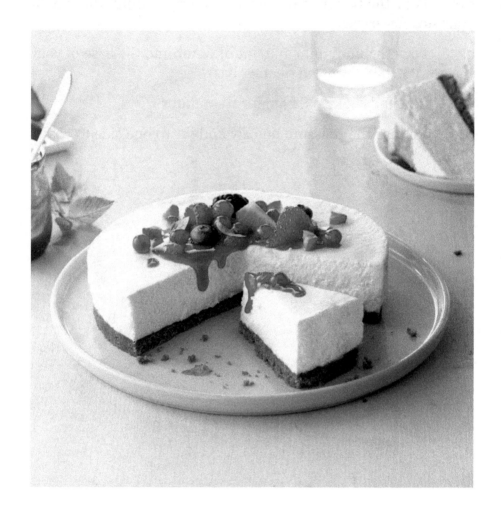

Preparation time: 45 minutes

Ingredients:

For the crust:

4 tbsp. butter

6 cups coconut, shredded

Any sweetener you consider appropriate

8 Oz. cream cheese

½ cup stevia sweetener

½ maple syrup

16 Oz. can of pineapple in a syrup, crashed or whole, drained

¼ cup whipping cream

5 eggs

Directions:

1.   After you mix all the crust ingredients press evenly and place it into the baking tray or pan and have it baked for at least 10 minutes. Let it cool.

2.   In a blender mix well the cream cheese with sweeteners, the pineapple until blended.

3.   Add the eggs gradually and pour this batter into the pan you have prepared.

4.   Bake for 90 minutes. Remove from oven and let it cooled.

Tip: Can be served with additional pineapple on top and/or with whipped cream whatever topping you choose to your liking.

Gluten-Free Nutella Brownie Trifle

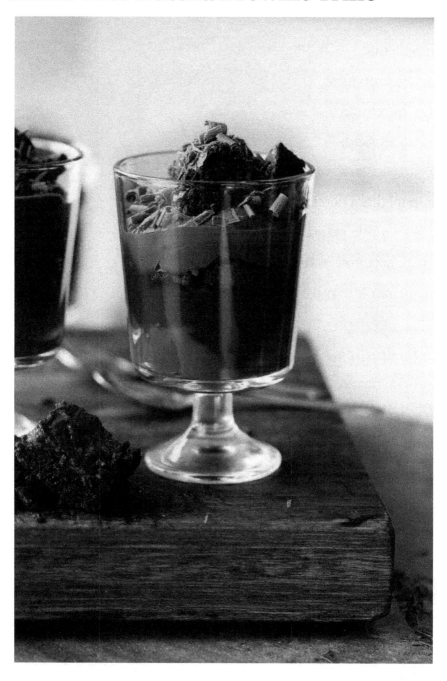

Preparation time: 60 minutes

Ingredients:

For the brownies:

6 Oz. hazelnuts

½ cup almonds

½ cup cashews

1 cup medjool dates, pitted

½ tsp. vanilla extract 2 tbsp. cacao powder

2 tbsp. hazelnut butter

1 tbsp. maple syrup or honey, to taste

For the frosting:

½ cup avocado, fresh crushed

1 ½ tbsp. coconut oil

½ tsp. vanilla

2tbsp. coconut maple syrup

1 tbsp. cacao

1 tbsp. nut butter

Directions:

1. You will need some baking paper for lining the baking tray.

2. Dry the hazelnuts and almonds in a frying pan until toasted.

3.   Add ¾ of all the nuts with the almonds into the food processor until they are broken to chunks.

4.   Add the dates and process again, then all the rest ingredients until you have a sticky mass.

5.   Pour it onto the baking tray lined with paper. Press the crumbly mixture you made with your fingers until the top of it is even. Place into the fridge while you are cooking the glaze.

6.   For the glaze you will have to mix well all the ingredients in a bowl or process them all in a food processor until well combined. It should be smooth and creamy.

7.   Remove your brownie from a fridge add the frosting on top spreading it evenly.

8.   Top the brownie with the remaining nuts and place again into the fridge until you have it served.

Low-Carb Curd Soufflé

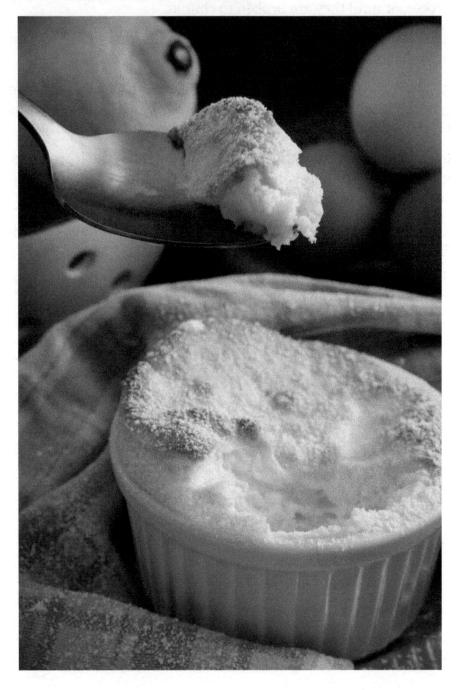

Preparation time: 45 minutes

Ingredients:

For the soufflé:

7 Oz. cream

½ cup condensed milk

1 pack (1 Oz.) gelatin for a dense soufflé

1 cup milk

5 Oz. cottage cheese

Directions:

1.   Fill the gelatin with milk and set aside.

2.   Mix the condensed milk with the cream and bring to boil on a low heat.

3.   Pour the gelatin mass into the boiled mixture and mix it, then let it cool.

4.   In a mixer, have all the mass combined well with the cottage cheese for at least 10 minutes.

5.   Pour it into the silicone moulds for the cupcakes and let it freeze for a couple of hours and serve.

Cream Cheese Cookies

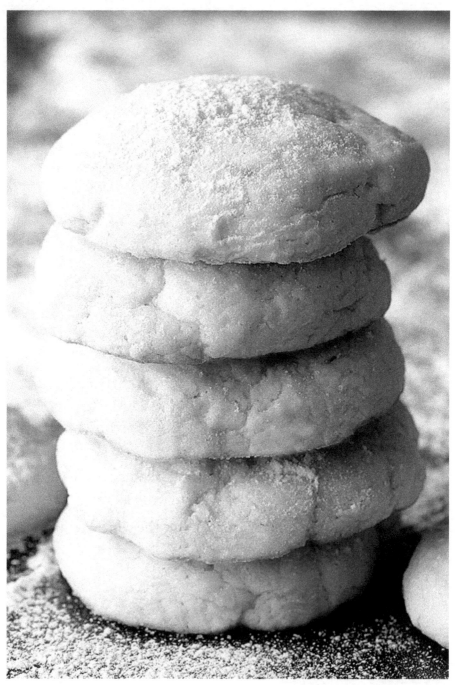

Preparation time: 40 minutes Ingredients:

1 cup butter

¾ cup stevia or any sugar substitute

4 Oz. cream cheese, softened

1   egg

2   cups almond flour

1 cup coconut flour

Sesame seeds

Vanilla or any flavored extract to taste

Directions:

1.   Mix the butter with the sweetener until fluffy.

2.   Beat the cream cheese and add the egg, then flour and mix it with the flavor and seeds you have chosen.

3.   Let it chill for 3-4 hours.

4.   Roll the cookie mass into a log and have it sliced thus forming your cookies.

5.   Bake until brown up to 15 minutes or more to make them crispy.

Chia Seeds Pudding with Berries

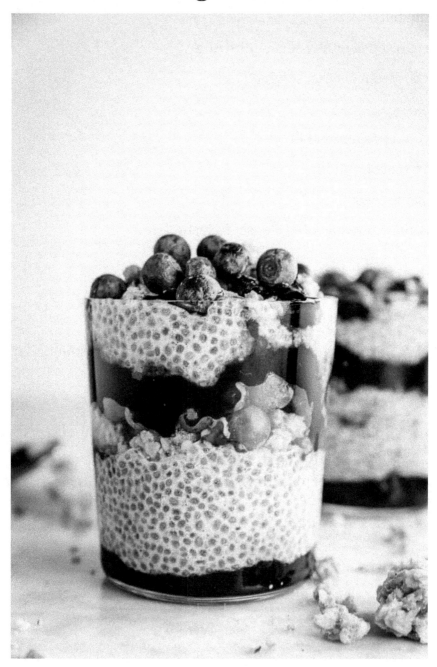

Preparation time: 60 minutes

Ingredients:

2 cups coconut milk, full fat

1 banana, sliced

½ cups chia seeds

Honey or stevia for sweetening

5 Oz. at least any fresh berries

Directions:

1.   Stir the milk, chia seeds and stevia (or honey) in a mixing bowl.

2.   Add half of all the berries and let the mixture chilled for at least 1 hour.

3.   Mix it up again and add the berries and banana before serving.

Tip: Chia seeds have omega-3 fatty acids, protein, fiber, calcium and antioxidants.

Smoothie Bowl

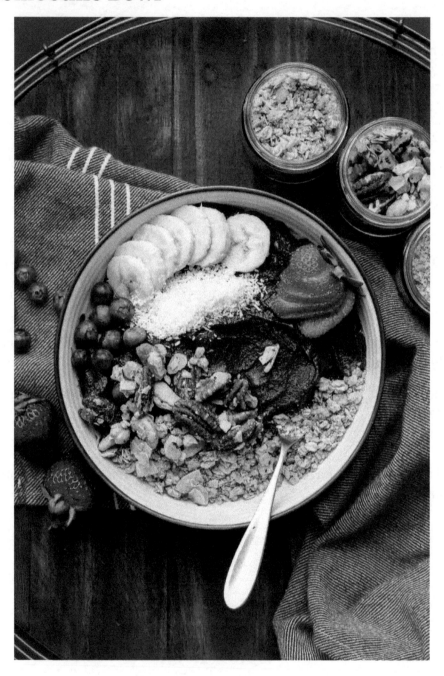

Preparation time: 45 minutes

Ingredients:

6 Oz. berries, fresh or frozen

2 medium frozen bananas

½ cup Almond milk

1 cup jellified yoghurt

1 tbsp. Chia seeds

1 tbsp. Hemp seeds

1 tbsp. Coconut flakes

Raspberry jam or any other, to taste

Directions:

1.   In a blender mix the bananas with half of the berries until it has a puree consistency.

2.   Organise your smoothie in a bowl decorating it in rows with the yogurt spot, the puree and fresh berries and with a pinch of seeds and flakes you have.

Coconut milk smoothie

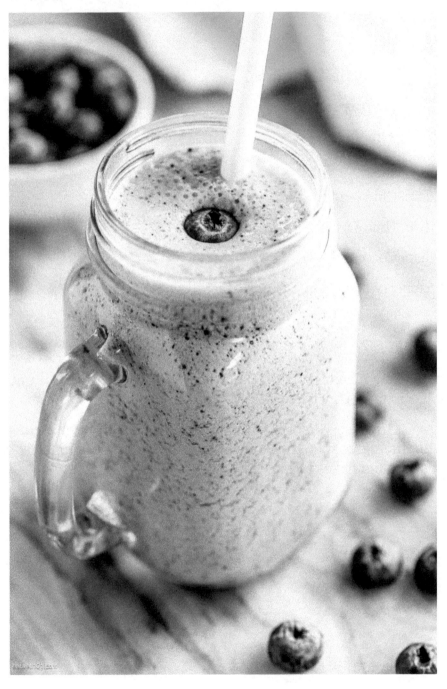

Preparation time: 15 minutes

Ingredients:

1 cup Greek yogurt

1 cup coconut milk, full fat

1 banana, fresh or frozen

1 cup baby spinach, fresh

1 tbsp. honey

5 Oz. blueberries or other berries

Directions:

1.   In a blender mix all the ingredients until smooth. Add the ice for a thicker smoothie.

Yogurt Smoothie with Cinnamon and Mango

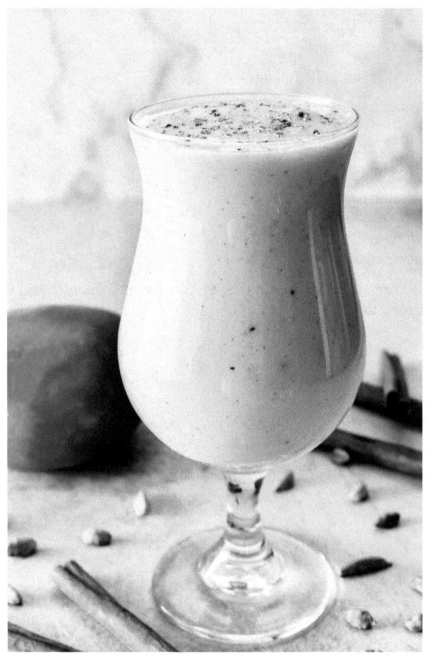

Preparation time: 15 minutes

Ingredients:

4 Oz. frozen mango chunks, mango pulp or fresh mango

1 cup Greek yogurt

1 cup coconut milk, full fat

3-4 cups milk

3 tbsp. flax seed meal

1 tbsp. honey

1   tsp. cinnamon

Directions:

1.   In a blender mix all the ingredients, except cinnamon until smooth. Sprinkle each smoothie with a pinch of cinnamon.

Lemon Curd Dessert (Sugar Free)

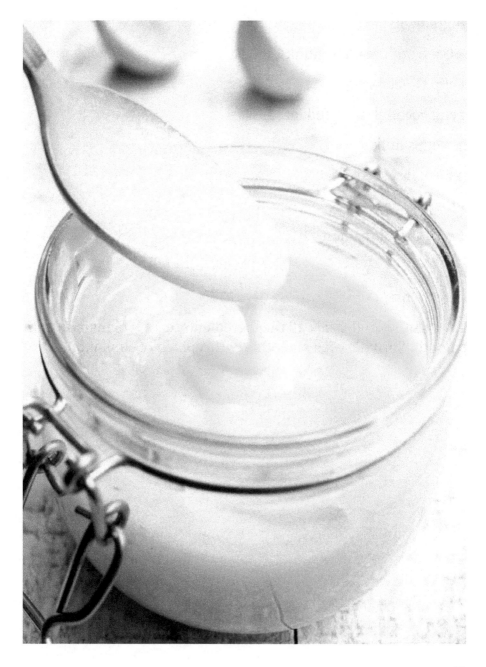

Preparation time: 35 minutes

Ingredients:

½ cup unsalted butter

½ cup lemon juice

2 tbsp. lemon zest

6 egg yolks

Stevia for sweetening

Directions:

1.   On a low heat melt the butter in a saucepan.

2.   Whisk in the stevia or any other sweetener, lemon ingredients until combined, then add the egg yolks and return to the stove again over the low heat.

3.   Whisk it until the curd starts thickening.

4.   Strain into a small bowl and let cool.

5.   Can be stored in a fridge for several weeks.

Chocolate Almond Butter Smoothie

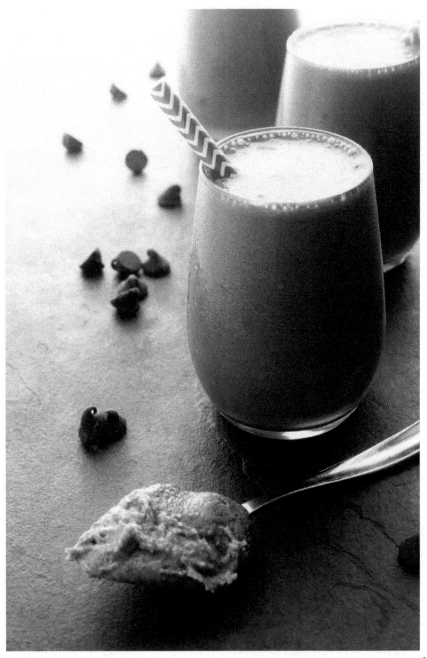

Preparation time: 35 minutes

Ingredients:

2   tbsp. chocolate protein powder

½ tbsp. cacao powder

1 cup almond milk

2 tbsp. almond butter

1 fresh banana

½ cup fresh strawberries

1 tbsp. chia or hemp seeds

Maple syrup or stevia for sweetening

Directions:

1.   Put all the ingredients into the blender and mix until it has creamy consistency.

Berry and Nuts Dessert

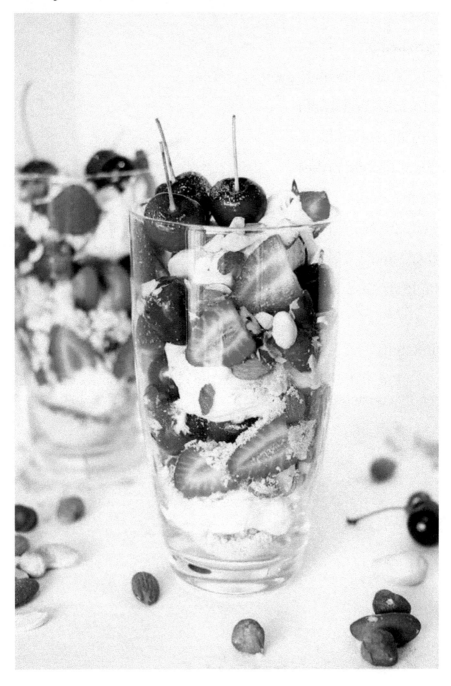

Preparation time: 25 minutes

Ingredients for 2 portions:

10 Oz. yogurt or yogurt drink

7 Oz. strawberries, fresh

Blueberries, raspberries or any berries you may like

1 banana, sliced

Pinch of Pistachio Pinch of cashews

4 walnuts, shelled

Pinch of pumpkin seeds

Pinch of sunflower seeds

Several fresh mint leaves

Directions:

1.   In a serving dish pour the jellied yogurt and top it with all the fresh ingredients.

Pastry with Nuts, Mango and Blueberries

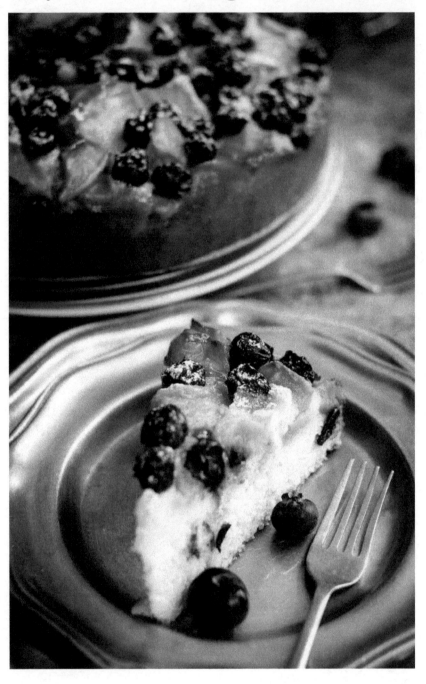

Preparation time: 45 minutes

Ingredients:

For the pastry:

1   cup whole wheat flour

½ cup whole wheat almond flour

½ cup butter

2 eggs yolks

2   Oz. water

12 Oz. blueberries or any berries to your liking

2 Mangoes

1 pinch of pumpkin seeds

Sesame and sunflower seeds

Peanuts, dried

For the filling:

8 Oz. cream cheese 1 mango, chopped

½ icing sugar

2 tbsp. lemon juice

Directions:

1.   In a bowl mix the flour ingredients with the butter, add the egg yolks and some water until combined and forms a ball.

2.   Knead the dough a little until it is smooth and refrigerate for half an hour covered with a napkin.

3.   Mix all the ingredients of the pastry filling in a blender.

4.   Grease your baking tray or a cooking tin and dust with some flour.

5.   Pour the dough into the tin and bake for 30 minutes (200 grades) until lightly brown.

6.   Pour the filling onto the pastry and top it with berries and nuts. Add some dessert sauce for serving.

Keto Vegan Pumpkin Mousse

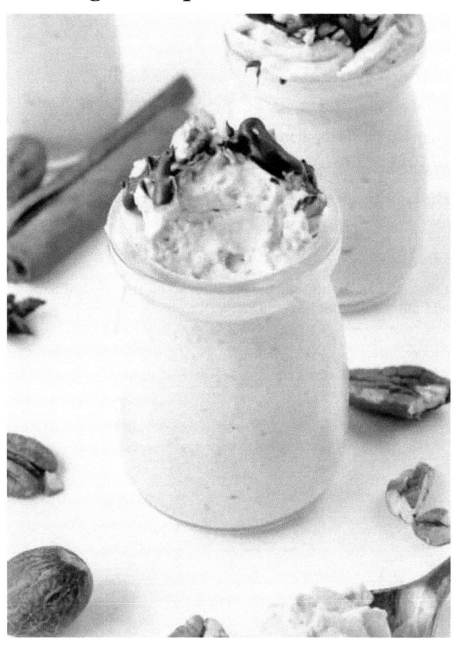

Preparation time: 15 minutes

Ingredients:

15 oz. firm Tofu

15 oz. organic

Pumpkin 1 tbsp. Cinnamon

½ tsp. Ginger

Stevia for sweetening

Directions:

1.   Mix all the ingredients in a blender until smooth. Taste and add more stevia for sweetening.

Keto Flax Seed Waffles

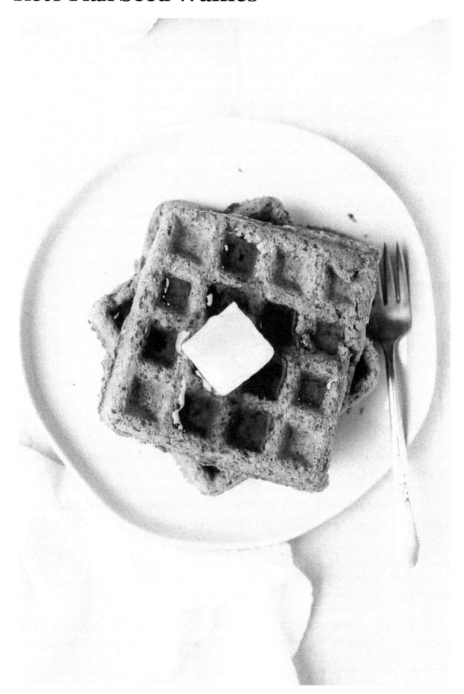

Preparation time: 20 minutes

Ingredients for 4 portions:

2 cups Golden Flax Seed

1 tbsp. Baking Powder

5 tbsp. Flax Seed Meal (mixed with 15 tbsp. Water)

⅓ cup Avocado Oil

½ cup Water 1 tsp.

Sea Salt

1 tbsp. fresh Herbs (thyme, rosemary or parsley) or 2 tsp. cinnamon, ground

Directions:

1.   Preheat the waffle-maker.

2.   Combine the flax seed with baking powder with a pinch of salt in a bowl. Whisk the mixture.

3.   Place the jelly-like flax seed mixture, some water and oil into the blender and pulse until foamy.

4.   Transfer the liquid mixture to the bowl with the flax seed mixture. Stir until combined. The mixture must be fluffy.

5.   Once it is combined, set aside for a couple of minutes. Add some fresh herbs or cinnamon. Divide the mixture into 4 servings.

6.   Scoop each, one at a time, onto the waffle maker. Cook with the closed top until it's ready. Repeat with the remaining batter.

7.   Eat immediately or keep in an air-tight container for a couple of weeks.

Keto Lemon Fat Bombs

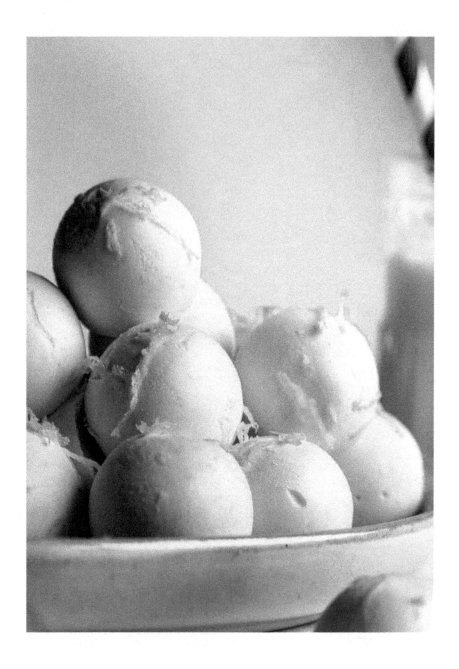

Preparation time: 60 minutes

Ingredients (for approx. 30 fat bombs):

1   cup Coconut Oil, melted

2   cups Raw Cashews, boiled for 10 minutes, soaked

½ cup Coconut Butter

1 Lemon Zest

2 Lemons, juiced

¼ cup Coconut Flour

⅓ cup Coconut, shredded

A pinch of salt

Stevia for sweetening

Directions:

1.   Mix all the ingredients in a food processor and blend until combined.

2.   Place the mixture to a bowl and have it cooled up in the freezer to 40 minutes.

3.   Remove from freezer and make the balls.

4.   Place them onto the cooking tray and again place into the freezer for hardening.

5.   Remove from the freezer and store in an air-tight container for up to a week. Let them thaw before serving.

Candied Pecans

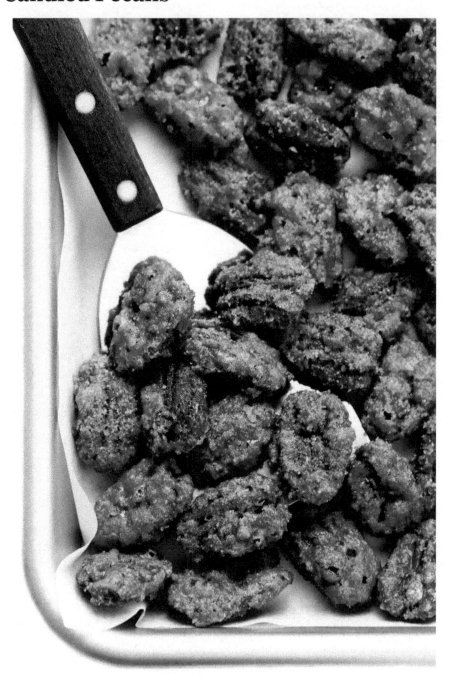

Preparation time: 60 minutes

Ingredients for 4 portions:

6 oz. Whole Pecans

½ cup Aquafaba

1 oz. Palm Sugar

1 oz. whole Green Cardamom Pods

¼ tsp. Salt

1   tsp. Allspice

Directions:

1.   Pre-heat oven to 350°F/180°C.

2.   Prepare a baking tray with a piece of parchment paper.

3.   Remove the cardamom seeds from the pods. Crush the seeds and lay them onto one side of the tray.

4.   Chop the sugar or grind it in a food processor.

5.   Whisk the aquafaba until frothy, stir in the sugar and salt. Fold in the nuts, allspice, cardamom, until everything is coated.

6.   Spread the mixture evenly over the baking tray for about 15 minutes and replace it onto the cooling rack.

7.   When cooled, pecans can be enjoyed as a topping or as they are.

Rice and Cantaloupe Ramekins

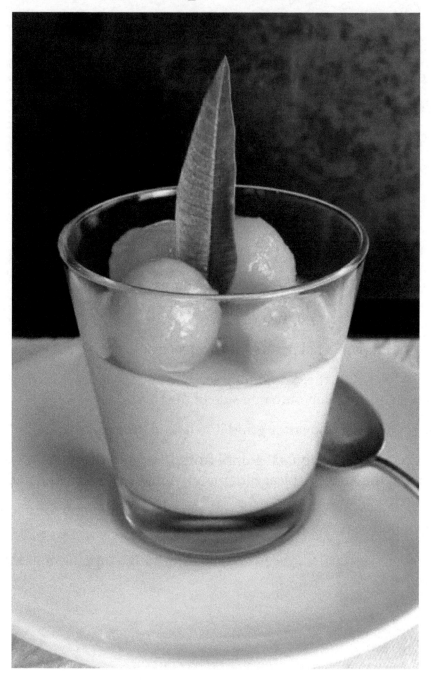

Preparation time: 10 minutes Cooking time: 30 minutes Servings: 4

Ingredients:

2   tablespoons flaxseed mixed with 3 tablespoons water

2 cups cauliflower rice, steamed

1 cup coconut cream

2 tablespoons stevia

1 teaspoon vanilla extract

½ cup cantaloupe, peeled and chopped

Cooking spray

Directions:

1.   In a bowl, mix the cauliflower rice with the flaxseed mix and the other ingredients except the cooking spray and whisk well.

2.   Grease 4 ramekins with the cooking spray, divide the rice mix in each and cook at 360 degrees F for 30 minutes.

3.   Serve cold.

Nutrition: calories 180, fat 5.3, fiber 5.4, carbs 11.5, protein 4

Strawberries Cream

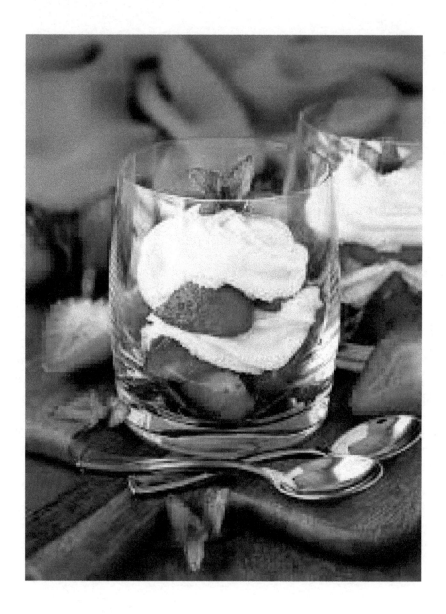

Preparation time: 10 minutes Cooking time: 0 minutes Servings: 2

Ingredients:

1 cup strawberries, chopped

1 cup coconut cream

1 tablespoon stevia

½ teaspoon vanilla extract

Directions:

1.   In a blender, combine the strawberries with the cream and the other ingredients, pulse well, divide into cups and serve cold.

Nutrition: calories 182, fat 3.1, fiber 2.3, carbs 3.5, protein 2

Almond and Chia Pudding

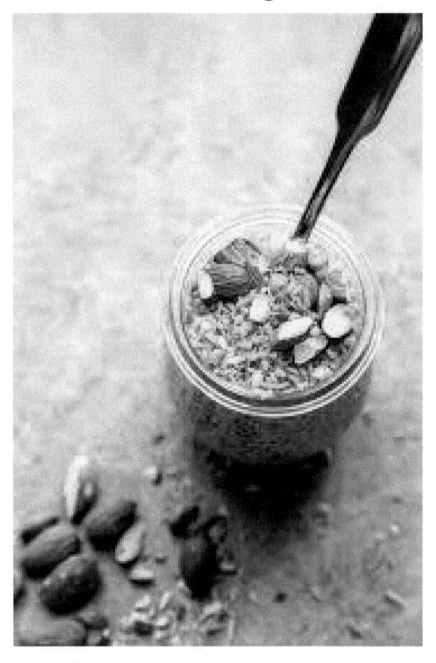

Preparation time: 10 minutes Cooking time: 15 minutes Servings: 4

Ingredients:

1 tablespoon lime juice

1   tablespoon lime zest, grated

2 cups almond milk

2   tablespoons almonds, chopped

1 teaspoon almond extract

½ cup chia seeds

2 tablespoons stevia

Directions:

1.   In a pan, mix the almond milk with the chia seeds, the almonds and the other ingredients, whisk, bring to a simmer and cook over medium heat for 15 minutes.

2.   Divide the mix into bowls and serve cold.

Nutrition: calories 174, fat 12.1, fiber 3.2, carbs 3.9, protein 4.8

Dates and Cocoa Bowls

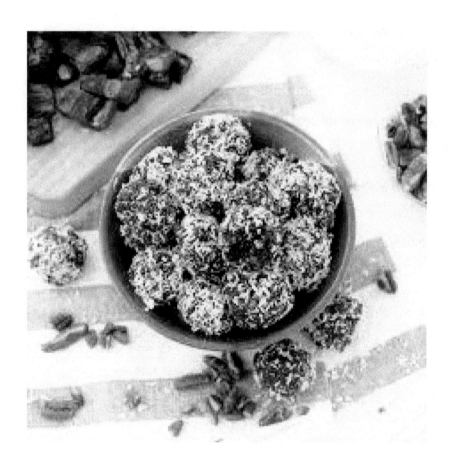

Preparation time: 2 hours Cooking time: 0 minutes Servings: 6

Ingredients:

2 tablespoons avocado oil

1 cup coconut cream

1 teaspoon cocoa powder

½ cup dates, chopped

3 tablespoons stevia

Directions:

1.   In a bowl, mix the cream with the oil, the cocoa, the cream and the other ingredients, pulse well, divide into cups and keep in the fridge for 2 hours before serving.

Nutrition: calories 141, fat 10.2, fiber 2.4, carbs 13.8, protein 1.4

Berries and Cherries Bowls

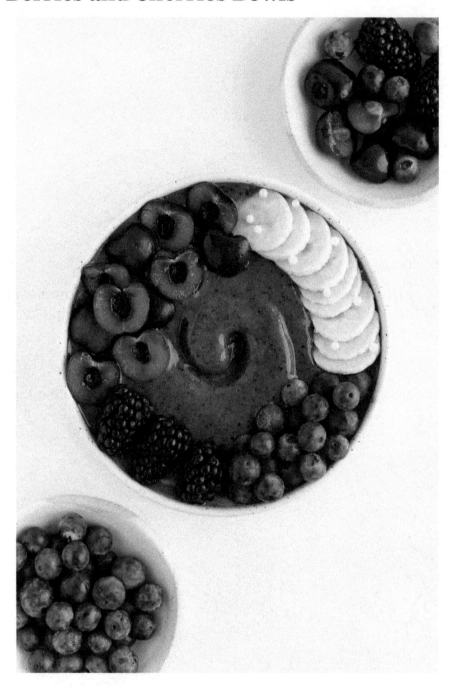

Preparation time: 10 minutes Cooking time: 0 minutes Servings: 4

Ingredients:

1 cup strawberries, halved

1 cup blackberries

1 cup cherries, pitted and halved

¼ cup coconut cream

¼ cup stevia

1   teaspoon vanilla extract

Directions:

1.   In a bowl, combine the berries with the cherries and the other ingredients, toss, divide into smaller bowls and serve cold.

Nutrition: calories 122, fat 4, fiber 5.3, carbs 6.6, protein 4.5

Cocoa Peach Cream

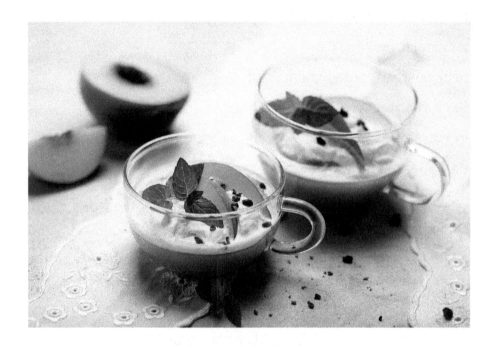

Preparation time: 10 minutes Cooking time: 0 minutes Servings: 4

Ingredients:

2   cups coconut cream

1/3 cup stevia

¾ cup cocoa powder

Zest of 1 lime, grated

1   tablespoons lime juice

2   peaches, pitted and chopped

Directions:

1.   In a blender, combine the cream with the stevia, the cocoa and the other ingredients, pulse well, divide into cups and serve cold.

Nutrition: calories 172, fat 5.6, fiber 3.5, carbs 7.6, protein 4

Nuts and Seeds Pudding

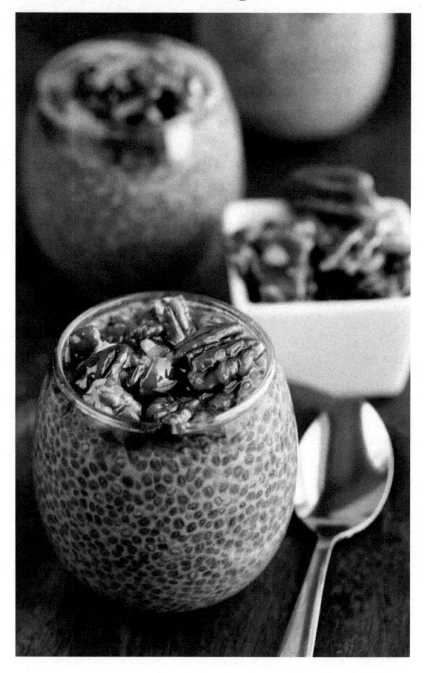

Preparation time: 10 minutes Cooking time: 20 minutes Servings: 4

Ingredients:

2 cups cauliflower rice

¼ cup coconut cream

2 cups almond milk

1 teaspoon vanilla extract

3 tablespoons stevia

½ cup walnuts, chopped

1 tablespoon chia seeds

Cooking spray

Directions:

1.   In a pan, combine the cauliflower rice with the cream, the almond milk and the other ingredients, toss, bring to a simmer and cook over medium heat for 20 minutes.

2.   Divide into bowls and serve cold.

Nutrition: calories 223, fat 8.1, fiber 3.4, carbs 7.6, protein 3.4

Cashew Fudge

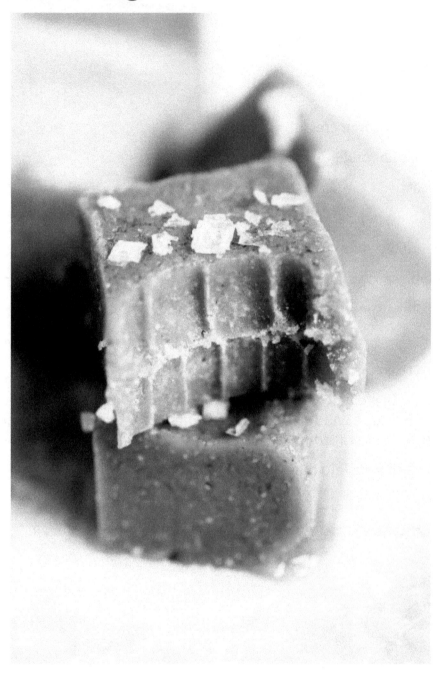

Preparation time: 3 hours Cooking time: 0 minutes Servings: 6

Ingredients:

1/3 cup cashew butter

1 cup coconut cream

½ cup cashews, soaked for

8 hours and drained

5 tablespoons lime juice

½ teaspoon lime zest, grated

1 tablespoons stevia

Directions:

1.   In a bowl, mix the cashew butter with the cream, the cashews and the other ingredients and whisk well.

2.   Line a muffin tray with parchment paper, scoop 1 tablespoon of the fudge mix in each of the muffin tins and freeze for 3 hours before serving.

Nutrition: calories 200, fat 4.5, fiber 3.4, carbs 13.5, protein 5

Lime Berries Stew

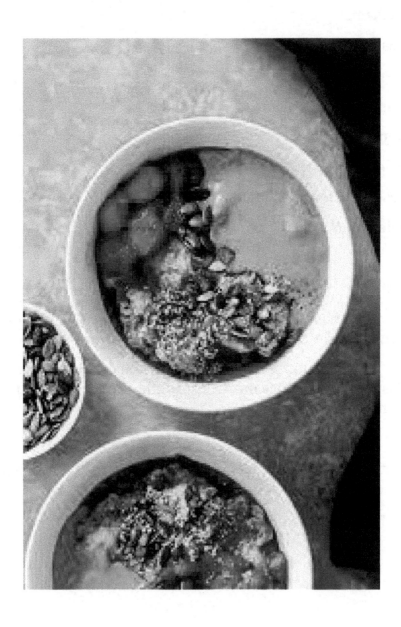

Preparation time: 10 minutes Cooking time: 20 minutes Servings: 6

Ingredients:

Zest of 1 lime, grated

Juice of 1 lime

1	pint strawberries, halved

2 cups water

2	tablespoons stevia

Directions:

1.	In a pan, combine the strawberries with the lime juice, the water and stevia, toss, bring to a simmer and cook over medium heat for 20 minutes.

2.	Divide the stew into bowls and serve cold.

Nutrition: calories 172, fat 7, fiber 3.4, carbs 8, protein 2.3

Apricots Cake

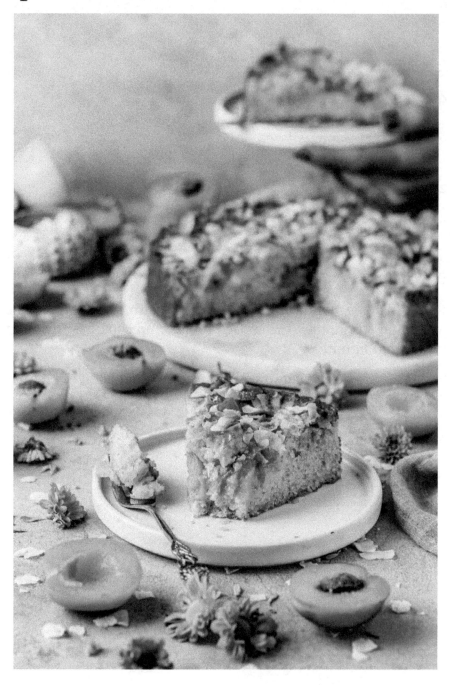

Preparation time: 10 minutes Cooking time: 30 minutes Servings: 8

Ingredients:

¾ cup stevia

2 cups coconut flour

¼ cup coconut oil, melted

½ cup almond milk

1   teaspoon baking powder

2   tablespoons flaxseed mixed with 3 tablespoons water

½ teaspoon vanilla extract

Juice of 1 lime

2 cups apricots, chopped

Directions:

1.   In a bowl, mix the flour with the coconut oil, the stevia and the other ingredients, whisk and pour into a cake pan lined with parchment paper.

2.   Introduce in the oven at 375 degrees F, bake for 30 minutes, cool down, slice and serve.

Nutrition: calories 221, fat 8.3, fiber 3.4, carbs 14.5, protein 5

Berry Cake

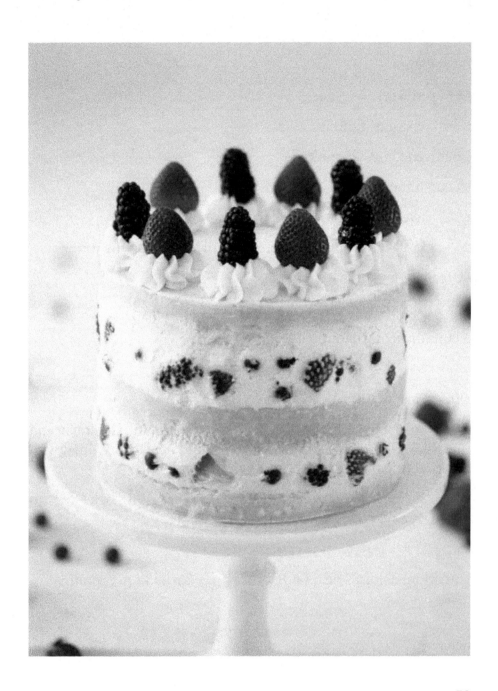

Preparation time: 10 minutes Cooking time: 30 minutes Servings: 6

Ingredients:

2 cups coconut flour

1 cup blueberries

1   cup strawberries, chopped

2   tablespoons almonds, chopped

2 tablespoons walnuts, chopped

3 tablespoons stevia

1 teaspoon almond extract

3 tablespoons flaxseed mixed with

4 tablespoons water

½ cup coconut cream

2 tablespoons avocado oil

1 teaspoon baking powder

Cooking spray

Directions:

1.   In a bowl, combine the coconut flour with the berries, the nuts, stevia and the other ingredients, and whisk well.

2.   Grease a cake pan with the cooking spray, pour the cake mix inside, introduce everything in the oven at 360 degrees F and bake for 30 minutes.

3.   Cool the cake down, slice and serve.

Nutrition: calories 225, fat 9, fiber 4.5, carbs 10.2, protein 4.5

Dates Mousse

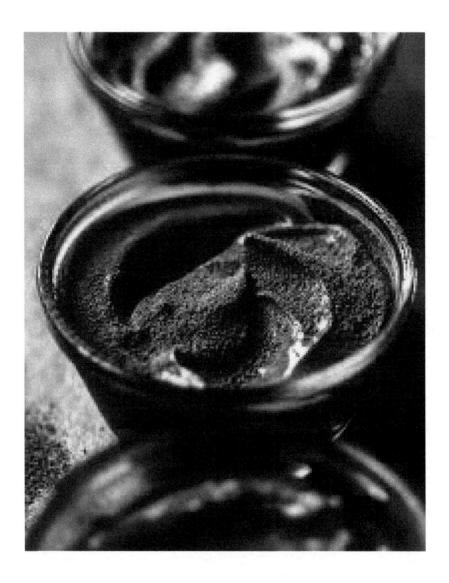

Preparation time: 30 minutes Cooking time: 0 minutes Servings: 4

Ingredients:

2 cups coconut cream

¼ cup stevia

2 cups dates, chopped

1 teaspoon almond extract

1 teaspoon vanilla extract

Directions:

1.   In a blender, combine the cream with the stevia, dates and the other ingredients, pulse well, divide into cups and keep in the fridge for 30 minutes before serving.

Nutrition: calories 141, fat 4.7, fiber 4.7, carbs 8.3, protein 0.8

Minty Almond Cups

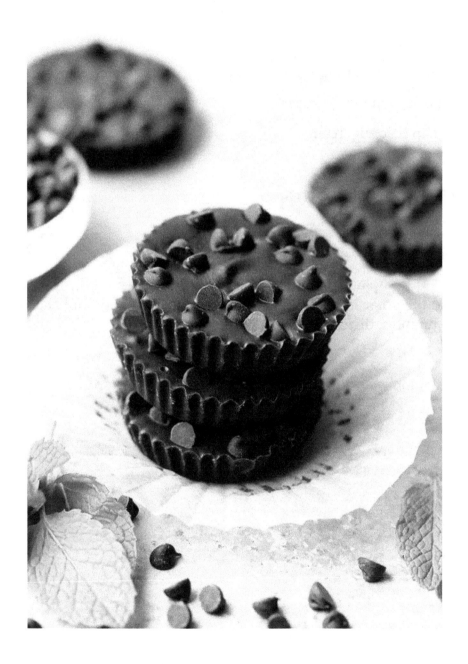

Preparation time: 10 minutes Cooking time: 10 minutes Servings: 4

Ingredients:

1 cup almonds, roughly chopped

1 tablespoon mint, chopped

½ cup coconut cream

2 tablespoons stevia

1 teaspoon vanilla extract

Directions:

1.   In a pan, combine the almonds with the mint, the cream and the other ingredients, whisk, simmer over medium heat for 10 minutes, divide into cups and serve cold.

Nutrition: calories 135, fat 4.1, fiber 3.8, carbs 4.1, protein 2.3

Lime Cake

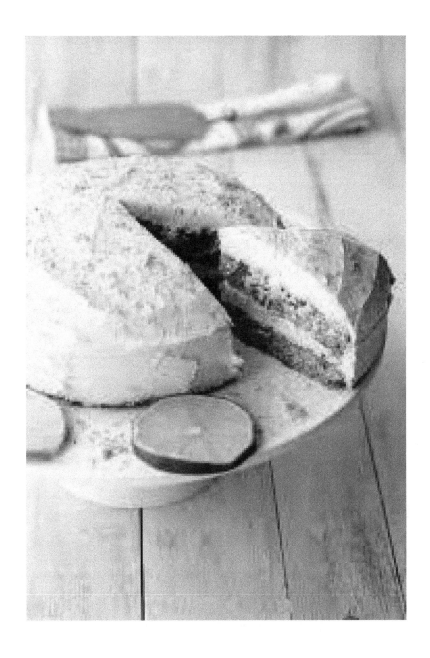

Preparation time: 10 minutes Cooking time: 40 minutes Servings: 4

Ingredients:

½ cup almonds, chopped

Zest of 1 lime grated

Juice of 1 lime

1   cups stevia

2   tablespoons flaxseed mixed with 3 tablespoons water

1 teaspoon vanilla extract

1 and ½ cup almond flour

½ cup coconut cream

1   teaspoon baking soda

Directions:

1.   In a bowl, combine the almond with the lime zest, lime juice and the other ingredients, whisk well and pour into a cake pan lined with parchment paper.

2.   Introduce in the oven at 360 degrees F, bake for 40 minutes, cool down, slice and serve.

Nutrition: calories 186, fat 16.4, fiber 3, carbs 6.8, protein 4.7

Vanilla Pudding

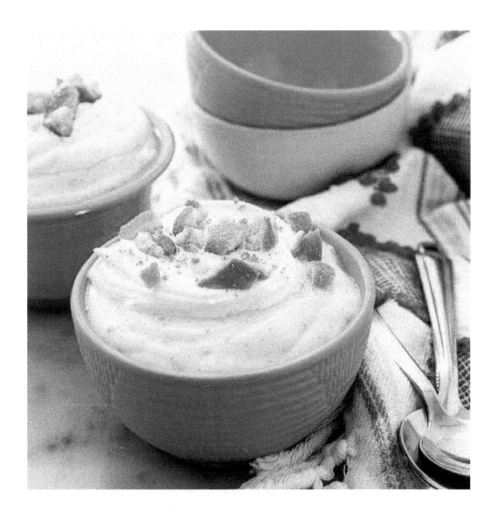

Preparation time: 10 minutes Cooking time: 40 minutes Servings: 4

Ingredients:

2   cups almond flour

3   tablespoons walnuts, chopped

1 and ½ cups coconut cream

3 tablespoons flaxseed mixed with 4 tablespoons water

1 cup stevia

1 teaspoon vanilla extract

1 teaspoon baking powder

1 teaspoon nutmeg, ground

Directions:

1.   In a bowl, combine the flour with the walnuts, the cream and the other ingredients, whisk well and pour into 4 ramekins.

2.   Introduce in the oven at 350 degrees F, bake for 40 minutes, cool down and serve.

Nutrition: calories 399, fat 39.3, fiber 4.7, carbs 11.2, protein 7.2

Cinnamon Avocado and Berries Mix

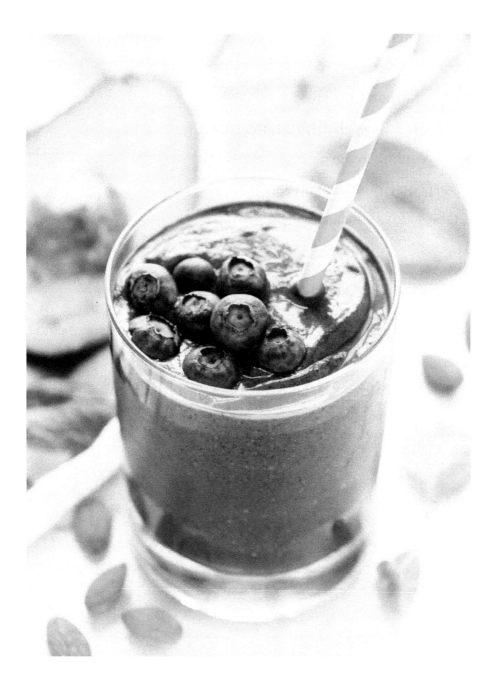

Preparation time: 5 minutes Cooking time: 0 minutes Servings: 4

Ingredients:

1 cup blackberries

1 cup strawberries, halved

1 cup avocado, peeled, pitted and cubed

1 cup coconut cream

1 teaspoon cinnamon powder

4 tablespoons stevia

Directions:

1.   In a bowl, combine the berries with the avocado and the other ingredients, toss, divide into smaller bowls and serve cold.

Nutrition: calories 162, fat 8, fiber 4.2, carbs 12.3, protein 8.4

Raisins and Berries Cream

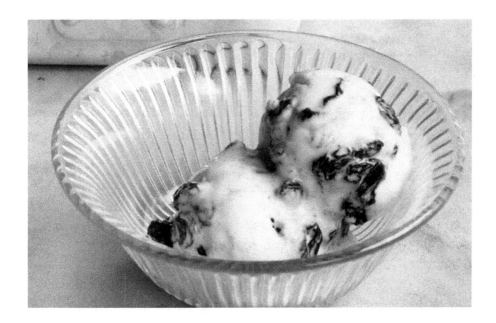

Preparation time: 5 minutes Cooking time: 0

Servings: 4

Ingredients:

1 cup coconut cream

1 cup blackberries

3 tablespoons stevia

2 tablespoons raisins

2 tablespoons lime juice

Directions:

1.   In a blender, the cream with the berries and the other ingredients except the raisins, pulse well, divide into cups, sprinkle the raisins on top and cool down before serving.

Nutrition: calories 192, fat 6.5, fiber 3.4, carbs 9.5, protein 5

Baked Rhubarb

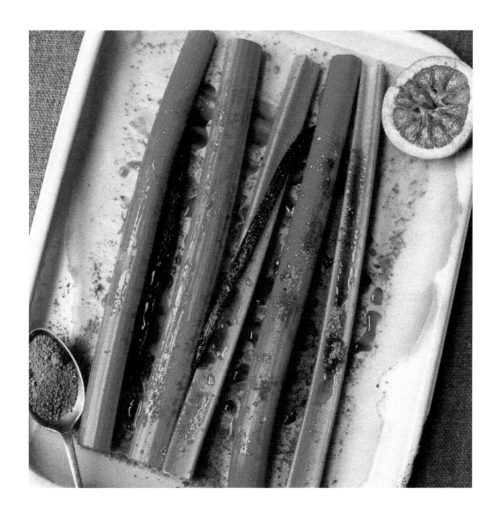

Preparation time: 10 minutes Cooking time: 20 minutes Servings: 4

Ingredients:

4 teaspoons stevia

1   pound rhubarb, roughly sliced

1 teaspoon vanilla extract

2   tablespoons avocado oil

1 teaspoon cinnamon powder

1 teaspoon nutmeg, ground

Directions:

1.   Arrange the rhubarb on a baking sheet lined with parchment paper, add the stevia, vanilla and the other ingredients, toss and bake at 350 degrees F for 20 minutes.

2.   Divide the baked rhubarb into bowls and serve cold.

Nutrition: calories 176, fat 4.5, fiber 7.6, carbs 11.5, protein 5

Cocoa Berries Mousse

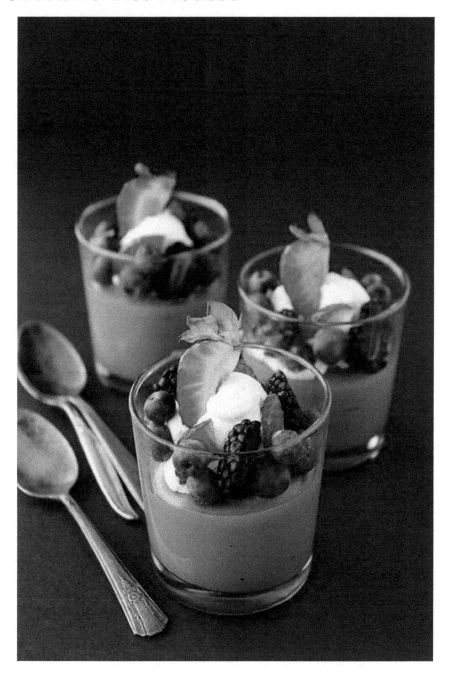

Preparation time: 10 minutes Cooking time: 0 minutes Servings: 2

Ingredients:

1 tablespoon cocoa powder

1 cup blackberries

1   cup blueberries

¾ cup coconut cream

1 tablespoon stevia

Directions:

1.   In a blender, combine the berries with the cocoa and the other ingredients, pulse well, divide into bowls and keep in the fridge for 2 hours before serving.

Nutrition: calories 200, fat 8, fiber 3.4, carbs 7.6, protein 4.3

Nutmeg Pudding

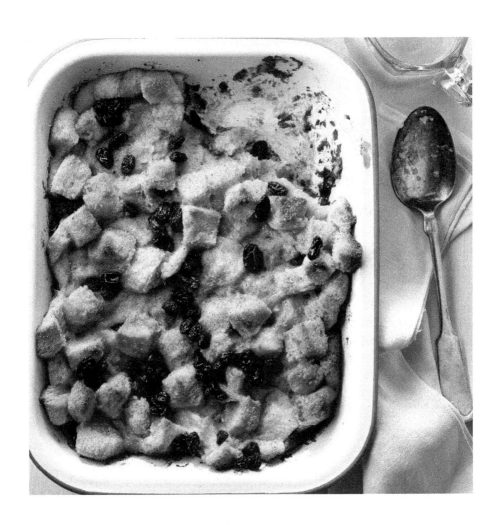

Preparation time: 10 minutes Cooking time: 20 minutes Servings: 6

Ingredients:

2   tablespoons stevia

1   teaspoon nutmeg, ground

1 cup cauliflower rice

2   tablespoons flaxseed mixed with 3 tablespoons water

2 cups almond milk

¼ teaspoon nutmeg, grated

Directions:

1.   In a pan, combine the cauliflower rice with the flaxseed mix and the other ingredients, whisk, cook over medium heat for 20 minutes, divide into bowls and serve cold.

Nutrition: calories 220, fat 6.6, fiber 3.4, carbs 12.4, protein 3.4

Lime Cherries and Rice Pudding

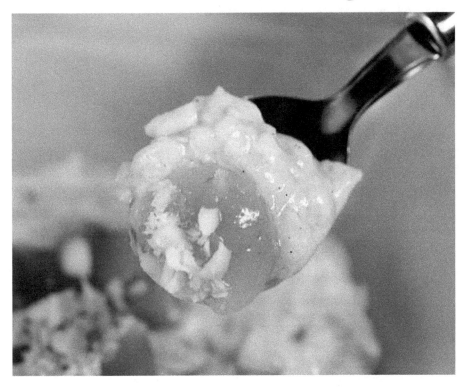

Preparation time: 10 minutes   Cooking time: 25 minutes
Servings: 4

Ingredients:

¾ cup stevia

2   cups coconut milk

3   tablespoons flaxseed mixed with 4 tablespoons water

Juice of 2 limes

Zest of 1 lime, grated

1   cup cherries, pitted and halved

1 cup cauliflower rice

Directions:

1.   In a pan, combine the milk with the stevia and bring to a simmer over medium heat.

2.   Add the cauliflower rice and the other ingredients, stir, cook for 25 minutes more, divide into cups and serve cold.

Nutrition: calories 199, fat 5.4, fiber 3.4, carbs 11.5, protein 5.6

Chocolate Pudding

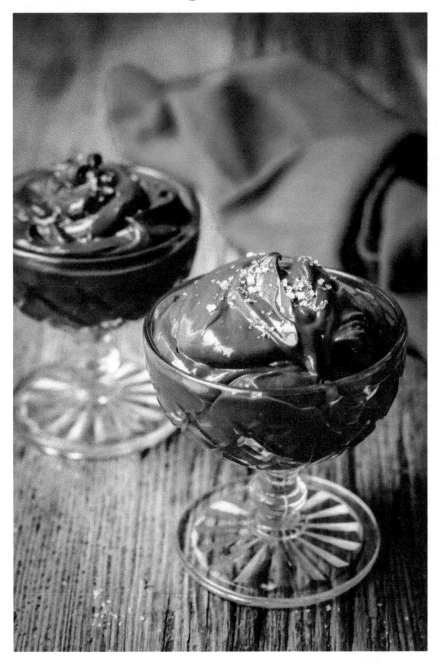

Preparation time: 10 minutes Cooking time: 20 minutes Servings: 4

Ingredients:

2   tablespoons cocoa powder

2 tablespoons coconut oil, melted 2/3 cup coconut cream

2 tablespoons stevia

¼ teaspoon almond extract

Directions:

1.   In a pan, combine the cocoa powder with the coconut milk and the other ingredients, whisk, bring to a simmer ad cook over medium heat for 20 minutes.

2.   Divide into cups and serve cold.

Nutrition: calories 134, fat 14.1, fiber 0.8, carbs 3.1, protein 0.9

Coffee and Rhubarb Cream

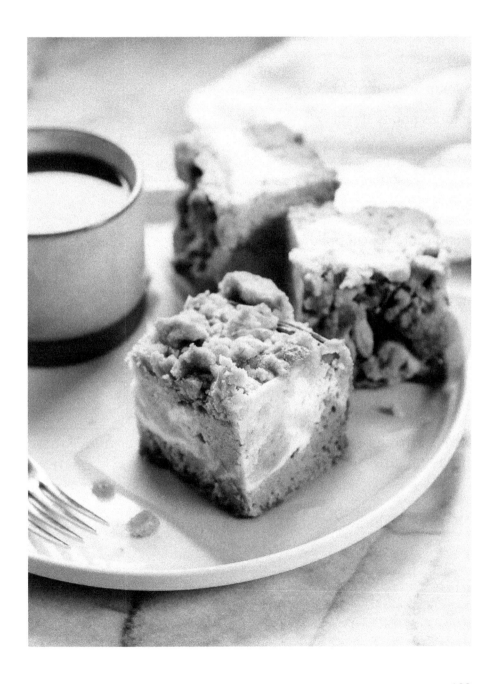

Preparation time: 10 minutes Cooking time: 20 minutes Servings: 4

Ingredients:

¼ cup brewed coffee

2 tablespoons stevia

2 cups coconut cream

1   teaspoon vanilla extract

2   tablespoons coconut oil, melted

1 cup rhubarb, chopped

2 tablespoons flaxseed mixed with 3

 tablespoons water

Directions:

1.   In a bowl, mix the coffee with stevia, cream and the other ingredients, whisk well and divide into 4 ramekins.

2.   Introduce the ramekins in the oven at 350 degrees F, bake for 20 minutes and serve warm.

Nutrition: calories 300, fat 30.8, fiber 0, carbs 3, protein 4

Avocado and Grapes Shake Bowls

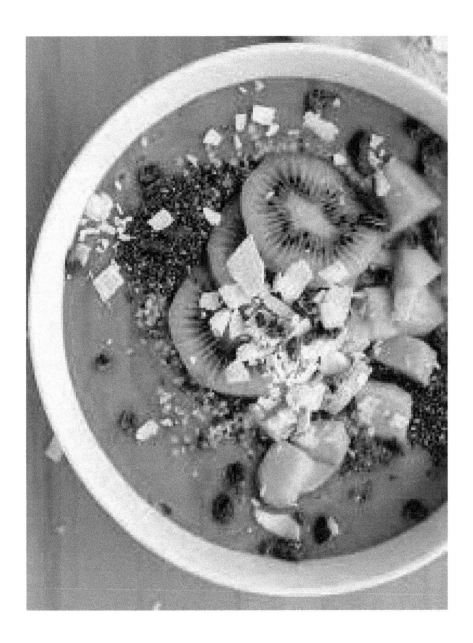

Preparation time: 5 minutes Cooking time: 0 minutes Servings: 4

Ingredients:

2 avocados, peeled, pitted and chopped

1 cup grapes, halved

Juice of 1 lime

¾ cup almond milk

½ teaspoon vanilla extract

Directions:

1.   In a blender, combine the avocados with the grapes and the other ingredients, pulse well, divide into bowls and serve cold.

Nutrition: calories 328, fat 30.4, fiber 8, carbs 16.1, protein 3.1

Chia Squares

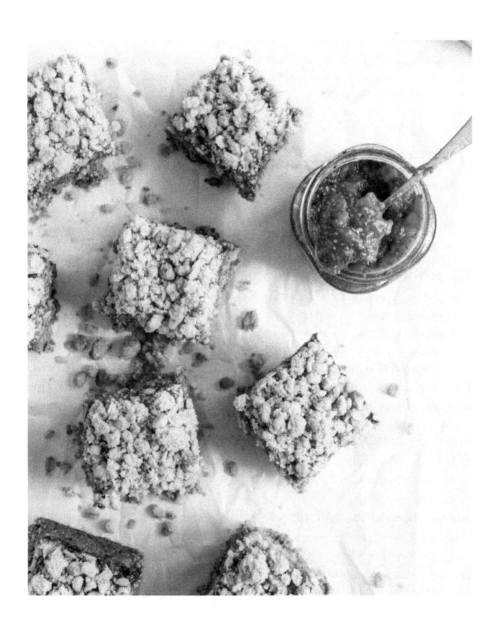

Preparation time: 30 minutes Cooking time: 0 minutes Servings: 4

Ingredients:

1   cup avocado oil

2   avocados, peeled, pitted and mashed

¼ cup coconut cream

1 tablespoon stevia

¼ cup lime juice

1 tablespoon chia seeds

A pinch of lemon zest, grated

Directions:

1.   In your food processor, combine the avocados with the oil, the cream and the other ingredients, pulse well and spread on the bottom of a pan.

2.   Introduce in the fridge for 30 minutes, slice into squares and serve.

Nutrition: calories 349, fat 32.5, fiber 12, carbs 15.8, protein 4.1

Blackberry Pie

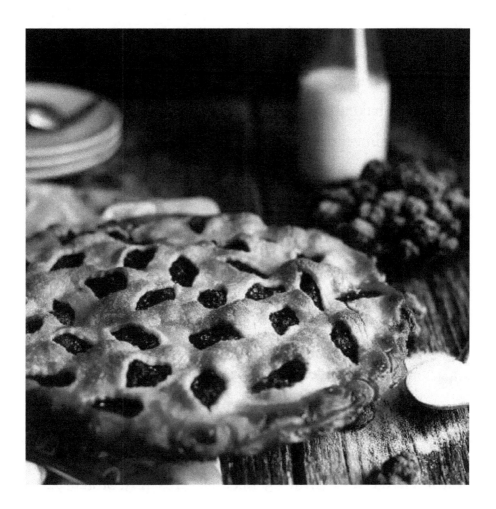

Preparation time: 10 minutes Cooking time: 35 minutes Servings: 6

Ingredients:

¾ cup stevia cups blackberries

¼ teaspoon baking soda

1 tablespoon lime juice

1 cup coconut flour

½ cup water

3 tablespoons avocado oil

 Cooking spray

Directions:

1.   In a bowl, combine the blackberries with the stevia, baking soda and the other ingredients, stir well and transfer to a pie pan.

2.   Introduce the pan in the oven at 375 degrees F, bake for 35 minutes, slice and serve warm.

Nutrition: calories 231, fat 5.5, fiber 24, carbs 42.3, protein 7.2

Lightning Source UK Ltd.
Milton Keynes UK
UKHW020653040521
383095UK00001B/67